This planner belongs to :

_____

2026

January

S	M	T	W	T	F	S
				1	2	3
4	5	6	7	8	9	10
11	12	13	14	15	16	17
18	19	20	21	22	23	24
25	26	27	28	29	30	31

February

S	M	T	W	T	F	S
1	2	3	4	5	6	7
8	9	10	11	12	13	14
15	16	17	18	19	20	21
22	23	24	25	26	27	28

March

S	M	T	W	T	F	S
1	2	3	4	5	6	7
8	9	10	11	12	13	14
15	16	17	18	19	20	21
22	23	24	25	26	27	28
29	30	31				

April

S	M	T	W	T	F	S
			1	2	3	4
5	6	7	8	9	10	11
12	13	14	15	16	17	18
19	20	21	22	23	24	25
26	27	28	29	30		

May

S	M	T	W	T	F	S
					1	2
3	4	5	6	7	8	9
10	11	12	13	14	15	16
17	18	19	20	21	22	23
24	25	26	27	28	29	30
31						

June

S	M	T	W	T	F	S
	1	2	3	4	5	6
7	8	9	10	11	12	13
14	15	16	17	18	19	20
21	22	23	24	25	26	27
28	29	30				

July

S	M	T	W	T	F	S
			1	2	3	4
5	6	7	8	9	10	11
12	13	14	15	16	17	18
19	20	21	22	23	24	25
26	27	28	29	30	31	

August

S	M	T	W	T	F	S
						1
2	3	4	5	6	7	8
9	10	11	12	13	14	15
16	17	18	19	20	21	22
23	24	25	26	27	28	29
30	31					

September

S	M	T	W	T	F	S
		1	2	3	4	5
6	7	8	9	10	11	12
13	14	15	16	17	18	19
20	21	22	23	24	25	26
27	28	29	30			

October

S	M	T	W	T	F	S
				1	2	3
4	5	6	7	8	9	10
11	12	13	14	15	16	17
18	19	20	21	22	23	24
25	26	27	28	29	30	31

November

S	M	T	W	T	F	S
1	2	3	4	5	6	7
8	9	10	11	12	13	14
15	16	17	18	19	20	21
22	23	24	25	26	27	28
29	30					

December

S	M	T	W	T	F	S
		1	2	3	4	5
6	7	8	9	10	11	12
13	14	15	16	17	18	19
20	21	22	23	24	25	26
27	28	29	30	31		

Year in Pixels

	J	F	M	A	M	J	J	A	S	O	N	D
1.												
2.												
3.												
4.												
5.												
6.												
7.												
8.												
9.												
10.												
11.												
12.												
13.												
14.												
15.												
16.												
17.												
18.												
19.												
20.												
21.												
22.												
23.												
24.												
25.												
26.												
27.												
28.												
29.												
30.												
31.												

Color Codes

Notes

January

MONDAY	TUESDAY	WEDNESDAY	THURSDAY
			1
5	6	7	8
12	13	14	15
19	20	21	22
26	27	28	29

January

FRIDAY	SATURDAY	SUNDAY	NOTES
2	3	4	○
			○
			○
			○
			○
9	10	11	○
			○
			○
			○
			○
16	17	18	○
			○
			○
			○
			○
23	24	25	○
			○
			○
			○
			○
30	31		NOTES

February

MONDAY	TUESDAY	WEDNESDAY	THURSDAY
2	3	4	5
9	10	11	12
16	17	18	19
23	24	25	26

February

2026

FRIDAY	SATURDAY	SUNDAY	NOTES
		1	○
			○
			○
			○
			○
6	7	8	○
			○
			○
			○
			○
13	14	15	○
			○
			○
			○
			○
20	21	22	○
			○
			○
			○
			○
27	28		NOTES

March

MONDAY	TUESDAY	WEDNESDAY	THURSDAY
2	3	4	5
9	10	11	12
16	17	18	19
23	24	25	26

March 2026

FRIDAY	SATURDAY	SUNDAY	NOTES
		1	○
			○
			○
			○
			○
6	7	8	○
			○
			○
			○
13	14	15	○
			○
			○
			○
			○
20	21	22	○
			○
			○
			○
			○
27	28	29	30 / 31

April 2026

MONDAY	TUESDAY	WEDNESDAY	THURSDAY
		1	2
6	7	8	9
13	14	15	16
20	21	22	23
27	28	29	30

April 2026

FRIDAY	SATURDAY	SUNDAY	NOTES
3	4	5	○
			○
			○
			○
			○
10	11	12	○
			○
			○
			○
			○
17	18	19	○
			○
			○
			○
24	25	26	○
			○
			○
			○
			○
			NOTES

May

MONDAY	TUESDAY	WEDNESDAY	THURSDAY
4	5	6	7
11	12	13	14
18	19	20	21
25	26	27	28

May

2026

FRIDAY	SATURDAY	SUNDAY	NOTES
1	2	3	○
			○
			○
			○
			○
8	9	10	○
			○
			○
			○
15	16	17	○
			○
			○
			○
			○
22	23	24	○
			○
			○
			○
			○
29	30	31	Notes

June

2026

MONDAY	TUESDAY	WEDNESDAY	THURSDAY
1	2	3	4
8	9	10	11
15	16	17	18
22	23	24	25
29	30		

June

2026

FRIDAY	SATURDAY	SUNDAY	NOTES
5	6	7	○
			○
			○
			○
			○
12	13	14	○
			○
			○
			○
19	20	21	○
			○
			○
			○
			○
26	27	28	○
			○
			○
			○
			○
			Notes

July

MONDAY	TUESDAY	WEDNESDAY	THURSDAY
		1	2
6	7	8	9
13	14	15	16
20	21	22	23
27	28	29	30

July

FRIDAY	SATURDAY	SUNDAY	NOTES
3	4	5	○
			○
			○
			○
			○
10	11	12	○
			○
			○
			○
			○
17	18	19	○
			○
			○
			○
24	25	26	○
			○
			○
			○
			○
31			NOTES

August 2026

MONDAY	TUESDAY	WEDNESDAY	THURSDAY
3	4	5	6
10	11	12	13
17	18	19	20
24	25	26	27

August

2026

FRIDAY	SATURDAY	SUNDAY	NOTES
	1	2	○
			○
			○
			○
			○
7	8	9	○
			○
			○
			○
			○
14	15	16	○
			○
			○
			○
			○
21	22	23	○
			○
			○
			○
			○
28	29	30	31

September

MONDAY	TUESDAY	WEDNESDAY	THURSDAY
	1	2	3
7	8	9	10
14	15	16	17
21	22	23	24
28	29	30	

September

2026

FRIDAY	SATURDAY	SUNDAY	NOTES
4	5	6	○
			○
			○
			○
			○
11	12	13	○
			○
			○
			○
			○
18	19	20	○
			○
			○
			○
25	26	27	○
			○
			○
			○
			○
			NOTES

October

MONDAY	TUESDAY	WEDNESDAY	THURSDAY
			1
5	6	7	8
12	13	14	15
19	20	21	22
26	27	28	29

October 2026

FRIDAY	SATURDAY	SUNDAY	NOTES
2	3	4	○
			○
			○
			○
			○
9	10	11	○
			○
			○
			○
			○
16	17	18	○
			○
			○
			○
23	24	25	○
			○
			○
			○
			○
30	31		NOTES

November 2026

MONDAY	TUESDAY	WEDNESDAY	THURSDAY
2	3	4	5
9	10	11	12
16	17	18	19
23	24	25	26

November

FRIDAY	SATURDAY	SUNDAY	NOTES
		1	○
			○
			○
			○
			○
6	7	8	○
			○
			○
			○
13	14	15	○
			○
			○
			○
			○
20	21	22	○
			○
			○
			○
			○
27	28	29	30

December

MONDAY	TUESDAY	WEDNESDAY	THURSDAY
	1	2	3
7	8	9	10
14	15	16	17
21	22	23	24
28	29	30	31

December
2026

FRIDAY	SATURDAY	SUNDAY	NOTES
4	5	6	○
			○
			○
			○
			○
11	12	13	○
			○
			○
			○
18	19	20	○
			○
			○
			○
			○
25	26	27	○
			○
			○
			○
			○
			NOTES

01 MONDAY

02 TUESDAY

03 WEDNESDAY

04 FRIDAY

05 FRIDAY

○ _____
○ _____
○ _____
○ _____
○ _____
○ _____
○ _____

06 SATURDAY

○ _____
○ _____
○ _____
○ _____
○ _____
○ _____
○ _____
○ _____

07 SUNDAY

○ _____
○ _____
○ _____
○ _____
○ _____
○ _____
○ _____
○ _____

08 MONDAY

○ _____
○ _____
○ _____
○ _____
○ _____

December
2025

09 TUESDAY

○ _____
○ _____
○ _____
○ _____
○ _____
○ _____
○ _____
○ _____

10 WEDNESDAY

○ _____
○ _____
○ _____
○ _____
○ _____
○ _____
○ _____
○ _____

11 THURSDAY

○ _____
○ _____
○ _____
○ _____
○ _____
○ _____
○ _____
○ _____

12 FRIDAY

○ _____
○ _____
○ _____
○ _____
○ _____

13 SATURDAY

14 SUNDAY

15 MONDAY

16 TUESDAY

17 WEDNESDAY

18 THURSDAY

19 FRIDAY

20 SATURDAY

21 SUNDAY

22 MONDAY

23 TUESDAY

24 WEDNESDAY

December
2025

25 THURSDAY

26 FRIDAY

27 SATURDAY

28 SUNDAY

December
2025

29 MONDAY

○
○
○
○
○
○
○
○

30 TUESDAY

○
○
○
○
○
○
○
○

31 WEDNESDAY

○
○
○
○
○
○
○
○

NOTES

01 THURSDAY

○
○
○
○
○
○
○
○

02 FRIDAY

○
○
○
○
○
○
○
○

03 SATURDAY

○
○
○
○
○
○
○
○

04 SUNDAY

○
○
○
○
○

05 MONDAY

○ _____
○ _____
○ _____
○ _____
○ _____
○ _____
○ _____

06 TUESDAY

○ _____
○ _____
○ _____
○ _____
○ _____
○ _____
○ _____
○ _____

07 WEDNESDAY

○ _____
○ _____
○ _____
○ _____
○ _____
○ _____
○ _____
○ _____

08 THURSDAY

○ _____
○ _____
○ _____
○ _____
○ _____

09 FRIDAY

○ _____
○ _____
○ _____
○ _____
○ _____
○ _____
○ _____
○ _____

10 SATURDAY

○ _____
○ _____
○ _____
○ _____
○ _____
○ _____
○ _____
○ _____

11 SUNDAY

○ _____
○ _____
○ _____
○ _____
○ _____
○ _____
○ _____
○ _____

12 MONDAY

○ _____
○ _____
○ _____
○ _____
○ _____

13 TUESDAY

14 WEDNESDAY

15 THURSDAY

16 FRIDAY

17 SATURDAY

○
○
○
○
○
○
○
○

18 SUNDAY

○
○
○
○
○
○
○
○

19 MONDAY

○
○
○
○
○
○
○
○

20 TUESDAY

○
○
○
○
○

21 WEDNESDAY

○ _____
○ _____
○ _____
○ _____
○ _____
○ _____
○ _____
○ _____

22 THURSDAY

○ _____
○ _____
○ _____
○ _____
○ _____
○ _____
○ _____
○ _____

23 FRIDAY

○ _____
○ _____
○ _____
○ _____
○ _____
○ _____
○ _____
○ _____

24 SATURDAY

○ _____
○ _____
○ _____
○ _____
○ _____

25 SUNDAY

○ _____
○ _____
○ _____
○ _____
○ _____
○ _____
○ _____
○ _____

26 MONDAY

○ _____
○ _____
○ _____
○ _____
○ _____
○ _____
○ _____
○ _____

27 TUESDAY

○ _____
○ _____
○ _____
○ _____
○ _____
○ _____
○ _____
○ _____

28 WEDNESDAY

○ _____
○ _____
○ _____
○ _____
○ _____

29 THURSDAY

○ _____
○ _____
○ _____
○ _____
○ _____
○ _____
○ _____
○ _____

30 FRIDAY

○ _____
○ _____
○ _____
○ _____
○ _____
○ _____
○ _____
○ _____

31 SATURDAY

○ _____
○ _____
○ _____
○ _____
○ _____
○ _____
○ _____
○ _____

NOTES

_____
_____
_____
_____

01 SUNDAY
○
○
○
○
○
○
○
○

02 MONDAY
○
○
○
○
○
○
○
○

03 TUESDAY
○
○
○
○
○
○
○
○

04 WEDNESDAY
○
○
○
○
○

05 THURSDAY

○ _____
○ _____
○ _____
○ _____
○ _____
○ _____
○ _____
○ _____

06 FRIDAY

○ _____
○ _____
○ _____
○ _____
○ _____
○ _____
○ _____
○ _____

07 SATURDAY

○ _____
○ _____
○ _____
○ _____
○ _____
○ _____
○ _____
○ _____

08 SUNDAY

○ _____
○ _____
○ _____
○ _____
○ _____

February 2026

09 MONDAY

○
○
○
○
○
○
○
○

10 TUESDAY

○
○
○
○
○
○
○
○

11 WEDNESDAY

○
○
○
○
○
○
○
○

12 THURSDAY

○
○
○
○
○

13 FRIDAY

14 SATURDAY

15 SUNDAY

16 MONDAY

17 TUESDAY
○
○
○
○
○
○
○
○

18 WEDNESDAY
○
○
○
○
○
○
○
○

19 THURSDAY
○
○
○
○
○
○
○
○

20 FRIDAY
○
○
○
○
○

21 SATURDAY

22 SUNDAY

23 MONDAY

24 TUESDAY

February
2026

25 WEDNESDAY
○
○
○
○
○
○
○
○

26 THURSDAY
○
○
○
○
○
○
○
○

27 FRIDAY
○
○
○
○
○
○
○
○

28 SATURDAY
○
○
○
○
○

March
2026

01 SUNDAY

○ _____
○ _____
○ _____
○ _____
○ _____
○ _____
○ _____
○ _____

02 MONDAY

○ _____
○ _____
○ _____
○ _____
○ _____
○ _____
○ _____
○ _____

03 TUESDAY

○ _____
○ _____
○ _____
○ _____
○ _____
○ _____
○ _____
○ _____

04 WEDNESDAY

○ _____
○ _____
○ _____
○ _____
○ _____

05 THURSDAY

○
○
○
○
○
○
○
○

06 FRIDAY

○
○
○
○
○
○
○
○

07 SATURDAY

○
○
○
○
○
○
○
○

08 SUNDAY

○
○
○
○
○

09 MONDAY

10 TUESDAY

11 WEDNESDAY

12 THURSDAY

13 FRIDAY

14 SATURDAY

15 SUNDAY

16 MONDAY

17 TUESDAY

18 WEDNESDAY

19 THURSDAY

20 FRIDAY

21 SATURDAY

22 SUNDAY

23 MONDAY

24 TUESDAY

25 WEDNESDAY

26 THURSDAY

27 FRIDAY

28 SATURDAY

March
2026

29 SUNDAY

○ _____
○ _____
○ _____
○ _____
○ _____
○ _____
○ _____

30 MONDAY

○ _____
○ _____
○ _____
○ _____
○ _____
○ _____
○ _____
○ _____

31 TUESDAY

○ _____
○ _____
○ _____
○ _____
○ _____
○ _____
○ _____
○ _____

NOTES

_____
_____
_____
_____

01 WEDNESDAY

02 THURSDAY

03 FRIDAY

04 SATURDAY

April
2026

05 SUNDAY

06 MONDAY

07 TUESDAY

08 WEDNESDAY

April
2026

09 THURSDAY

10 FRIDAY

11 SATURDAY

12 SUNDAY

13 MONDAY

14 TUESDAY

15 WEDNESDAY

16 THURSDAY

April
2026

17 FRIDAY

18 SATURDAY

19 SUNDAY

20 MONDAY

21 TUESDAY

22 WEDNESDAY

23 THURSDAY

24 FRIDAY

25 SATURDAY

26 SUNDAY

27 MONDAY

28 TUESDAY

29 WEDNESDAY

30 THURSDAY

NOTES

May
2026

01 FRIDAY

○ _____
○ _____
○ _____
○ _____
○ _____
○ _____
○ _____

02 SATURDAY

○ _____
○ _____
○ _____
○ _____
○ _____
○ _____
○ _____
○ _____

03 SUNDAY

○ _____
○ _____
○ _____
○ _____
○ _____
○ _____
○ _____
○ _____

04 MONDAY

○ _____
○ _____
○ _____
○ _____
○ _____

May
2026

05 TUESDAY

06 WEDNESDAY

07 THURSDAY

08 FRIDAY

09 SATURDAY

10 SUNDAY

11 MONDAY

12 TUESDAY

13 WEDNESDAY

14 THURSDAY

15 FRIDAY

16 SATURDAY

17 SUNDAY

18 MONDAY

19 TUESDAY

20 WEDNESDAY

21 THURSDAY

22 FRIDAY

23 SATURDAY

24 SUNDAY

25 MONDAY

26 TUESDAY

27 WEDNESDAY

28 THURSDAY

May
2026

29 FRIDAY

○ _____
○ _____
○ _____
○ _____
○ _____
○ _____
○ _____
○ _____

30 SATURDAY

○ _____
○ _____
○ _____
○ _____
○ _____
○ _____
○ _____
○ _____

31 SUNDAY

○ _____
○ _____
○ _____
○ _____
○ _____
○ _____
○ _____
○ _____

NOTES

_____
_____
_____
_____
_____

01 MONDAY

○ _____
○ _____
○ _____
○ _____
○ _____
○ _____
○ _____
○ _____

02 TUESDAY

○ _____
○ _____
○ _____
○ _____
○ _____
○ _____
○ _____
○ _____

03 WEDNESDAY

○ _____
○ _____
○ _____
○ _____
○ _____
○ _____
○ _____
○ _____

04 THURSDAY

○ _____
○ _____
○ _____
○ _____
○ _____

05 FRIDAY

06 SATURDAY

07 SUNDAY

08 MONDAY

09 TUESDAY

○ _____
○ _____
○ _____
○ _____
○ _____
○ _____
○ _____

10 WEDNESDAY

○ _____
○ _____
○ _____
○ _____
○ _____
○ _____
○ _____
○ _____

11 THURSDAY

○ _____
○ _____
○ _____
○ _____
○ _____
○ _____
○ _____
○ _____

12 FRIDAY

○ _____
○ _____
○ _____
○ _____
○ _____

13 SATURDAY

14 SUNDAY

15 MONDAY

16 TUESDAY

17 WEDNESDAY

○ _____
○ _____
○ _____
○ _____
○ _____
○ _____
○ _____
○ _____

18 THURSDAY

○ _____
○ _____
○ _____
○ _____
○ _____
○ _____
○ _____
○ _____

19 FRIDAY

○ _____
○ _____
○ _____
○ _____
○ _____
○ _____
○ _____
○ _____

20 SATURDAY

○ _____
○ _____
○ _____
○ _____
○ _____

June
2026

21 SUNDAY

○
○
○
○
○
○
○
○

22 MONDAY

○
○
○
○
○
○
○
○

23 TUESDAY

○
○
○
○
○
○
○
○

24 WEDNESDAY

○
○
○
○
○

25 THURSDAY

○ _____
○ _____
○ _____
○ _____
○ _____
○ _____
○ _____
○ _____

26 FRIDAY

○ _____
○ _____
○ _____
○ _____
○ _____
○ _____
○ _____
○ _____

27 SATURDAY

○ _____
○ _____
○ _____
○ _____
○ _____
○ _____
○ _____
○ _____

28 SUNDAY

○ _____
○ _____
○ _____
○ _____
○ _____

29 MONDAY

○
○
○
○
○
○
○
○

30 TUESDAY

○
○
○
○
○
○
○
○

NOTES

01 WEDNESDAY

○ _____
○ _____
○ _____
○ _____
○ _____
○ _____
○ _____
○ _____

02 THURSDAY

○ _____
○ _____
○ _____
○ _____
○ _____
○ _____
○ _____
○ _____

03 FRIDAY

○ _____
○ _____
○ _____
○ _____
○ _____
○ _____
○ _____
○ _____

04 SATURDAY

○ _____
○ _____
○ _____
○ _____
○ _____

05 SUNDAY

○
○
○
○
○
○
○
○

06 MONDAY

○
○
○
○
○
○
○
○

07 TUESDAY

○
○
○
○
○
○
○
○

08 WEDNESDAY

○
○
○
○
○

09 THURSDAY

10 FRIDAY

11 SATURDAY

12 SUNDAY

13 MONDAY

○ _____
○ _____
○ _____
○ _____
○ _____
○ _____
○ _____
○ _____

14 TUESDAY

○ _____
○ _____
○ _____
○ _____
○ _____
○ _____
○ _____
○ _____

15 WEDNESDAY

○ _____
○ _____
○ _____
○ _____
○ _____
○ _____
○ _____
○ _____

16 THURSDAY

○ _____
○ _____
○ _____
○ _____
○ _____

July
2026

17 FRIDAY

18 SATURDAY

19 SUNDAY

20 MONDAY

21 TUESDAY

○
○
○
○
○
○
○
○

22 WEDNESDAY

○
○
○
○
○
○
○
○

23 THURSDAY

○
○
○
○
○
○
○
○

24 FRIDAY

○
○
○
○
○

25 SATURDAY

26 SUNDAY

27 MONDAY

28 TUESDAY

July
2026

29 WEDNESDAY

30 THURSDAY

31 FRIDAY

NOTES

August
2026

01 SATURDAY

○ _____
○ _____
○ _____
○ _____
○ _____
○ _____
○ _____
○ _____

02 SUNDAY

○ _____
○ _____
○ _____
○ _____
○ _____
○ _____
○ _____
○ _____

03 MONDAY

○ _____
○ _____
○ _____
○ _____
○ _____
○ _____
○ _____
○ _____

04 TUESDAY

○ _____
○ _____
○ _____
○ _____
○ _____

05 WEDNESDAY

○ _____
○ _____
○ _____
○ _____
○ _____
○ _____
○ _____
○ _____

06 THURSDAY

○ _____
○ _____
○ _____
○ _____
○ _____
○ _____
○ _____
○ _____

07 FRIDAY

○ _____
○ _____
○ _____
○ _____
○ _____
○ _____
○ _____
○ _____

08 SATURDAY

○ _____
○ _____
○ _____
○ _____
○ _____

August
2026

09 SUNDAY

10 MONDAY

11 TUESDAY

12 WEDNESDAY

13 THURSDAY

14 FRIDAY

15 SATURDAY

16 SUNDAY

17 MONDAY

18 TUESDAY

19 WEDNESDAY

20 THURSDAY

21 FRIDAY

22 SATURDAY

23 SUNDAY

24 MONDAY

25 TUESDAY

26 WEDNESDAY

27 THURSDAY

28 FRIDAY

29 SATURDAY

30 SUNDAY

31 MONDAY

NOTES

01 TUESDAY

- ○
- ○
- ○
- ○
- ○
- ○
- ○
- ○

02 WEDNESDAY

- ○
- ○
- ○
- ○
- ○
- ○
- ○
- ○

03 THURSDAY

- ○
- ○
- ○
- ○
- ○
- ○
- ○
- ○

04 FRIDAY

- ○
- ○
- ○
- ○
- ○

05 SATURDAY

- ○
- ○
- ○
- ○
- ○
- ○
- ○
- ○

06 SUNDAY

- ○
- ○
- ○
- ○
- ○
- ○
- ○
- ○

07 MONDAY

- ○
- ○
- ○
- ○
- ○
- ○
- ○
- ○

08 TUESDAY

- ○
- ○
- ○
- ○
- ○

09 WEDNESDAY

○ _____
○ _____
○ _____
○ _____
○ _____
○ _____
○ _____
○ _____

10 THURSDAY

○ _____
○ _____
○ _____
○ _____
○ _____
○ _____
○ _____
○ _____

11 FRIDAY

○ _____
○ _____
○ _____
○ _____
○ _____
○ _____
○ _____
○ _____

12 SATURDAY

○ _____
○ _____
○ _____
○ _____
○ _____

13 SUNDAY

○ _____
○ _____
○ _____
○ _____
○ _____
○ _____
○ _____
○ _____

14 MONDAY

○ _____
○ _____
○ _____
○ _____
○ _____
○ _____
○ _____
○ _____

15 TUESDAY

○ _____
○ _____
○ _____
○ _____
○ _____
○ _____
○ _____
○ _____

16 WEDNESDAY

○ _____
○ _____
○ _____
○ _____
○ _____

17 THURSDAY

- ○
- ○
- ○
- ○
- ○
- ○
- ○
- ○

18 FRIDAY

- ○
- ○
- ○
- ○
- ○
- ○
- ○
- ○

19 SATURDAY

- ○
- ○
- ○
- ○
- ○
- ○
- ○
- ○

20 SUNDAY

- ○
- ○
- ○
- ○
- ○

21 MONDAY

○
○
○
○
○
○
○
○

22 TUESDAY

○
○
○
○
○
○
○
○

23 WEDNESDAY

○
○
○
○
○
○
○
○

24 THURSDAY

○
○
○
○
○

25 FRIDAY

○ _____
○ _____
○ _____
○ _____
○ _____
○ _____
○ _____
○ _____

26 SATURDAY

○ _____
○ _____
○ _____
○ _____
○ _____
○ _____
○ _____
○ _____
○ _____

27 SUNDAY

○ _____
○ _____
○ _____
○ _____
○ _____
○ _____
○ _____
○ _____

28 MONDAY

○ _____
○ _____
○ _____
○ _____
○ _____

29 TUESDAY

○ _____
○ _____
○ _____
○ _____
○ _____
○ _____
○ _____
○ _____

30 WEDNESDAY

○ _____
○ _____
○ _____
○ _____
○ _____
○ _____
○ _____
○ _____

NOTES

_____
_____
_____
_____
_____
_____
_____
_____
_____
_____
_____
_____
_____

October
2026

01 THURSDAY

02 FRIDAY

03 SATURDAY

04 SUNDAY

October
2026

05 MONDAY

○
○
○
○
○
○
○

06 TUESDAY

○
○
○
○
○
○
○

07 WEDNESDAY

○
○
○
○
○
○
○

08 THURSDAY

○
○
○
○

09 FRIDAY

10 SATURDAY

11 SUNDAY

12 MONDAY

13 TUESDAY

14 WEDNESDAY

15 THURSDAY

16 FRIDAY

October
2026

17 SATURDAY

18 SUNDAY

19 MONDAY

20 TUESDAY

October
2026

21 WEDNESDAY

22 THURSDAY

23 FRIDAY

24 SATURDAY

October
2026

25 SUNDAY

○
○
○
○
○
○
○
○

26 MONDAY

○
○
○
○
○
○
○
○

27 TUESDAY

○
○
○
○
○
○
○
○

28 WEDNESDAY

○
○
○
○
○

October
2026

29 THURSDAY

30 FRIDAY

31 SATURDAY

NOTES

November
2026

01 SUNDAY

02 MONDAY

03 TUESDAY

04 WEDNESDAY

November
2026

05 THURSDAY

06 FRIDAY

07 SATURDAY

08 SUNDAY

09 MONDAY

10 TUESDAY

11 WEDNESDAY

12 THURSDAY

13 FRIDAY

○ _____
○ _____
○ _____
○ _____
○ _____
○ _____
○ _____
○ _____

14 SATURDAY

○ _____
○ _____
○ _____
○ _____
○ _____
○ _____
○ _____
○ _____

15 SUNDAY

○ _____
○ _____
○ _____
○ _____
○ _____
○ _____
○ _____
○ _____

16 MONDAY

○ _____
○ _____
○ _____
○ _____
○ _____

17 TUESDAY

18 WEDNESDAY

19 THURSDAY

20 FRIDAY

21 SATURDAY

○
○
○
○
○
○
○
○

22 SUNDAY

○
○
○
○
○
○
○
○

23 MONDAY

○
○
○
○
○
○
○
○

24 TUESDAY

○
○
○
○
○

25 WEDNESDAY

26 THURSDAY

27 FRIDAY

28 SATURDAY

29 SUNDAY

○ _____
○ _____
○ _____
○ _____
○ _____
○ _____
○ _____
○ _____

30 MONDAY

○ _____
○ _____
○ _____
○ _____
○ _____
○ _____
○ _____
○ _____

NOTES

_____
_____
_____
_____
_____
_____
_____
_____
_____
_____
_____
_____
_____

December
2026

01 TUESDAY

02 WEDNESDAY

03 THURSDAY

04 FRIDAY

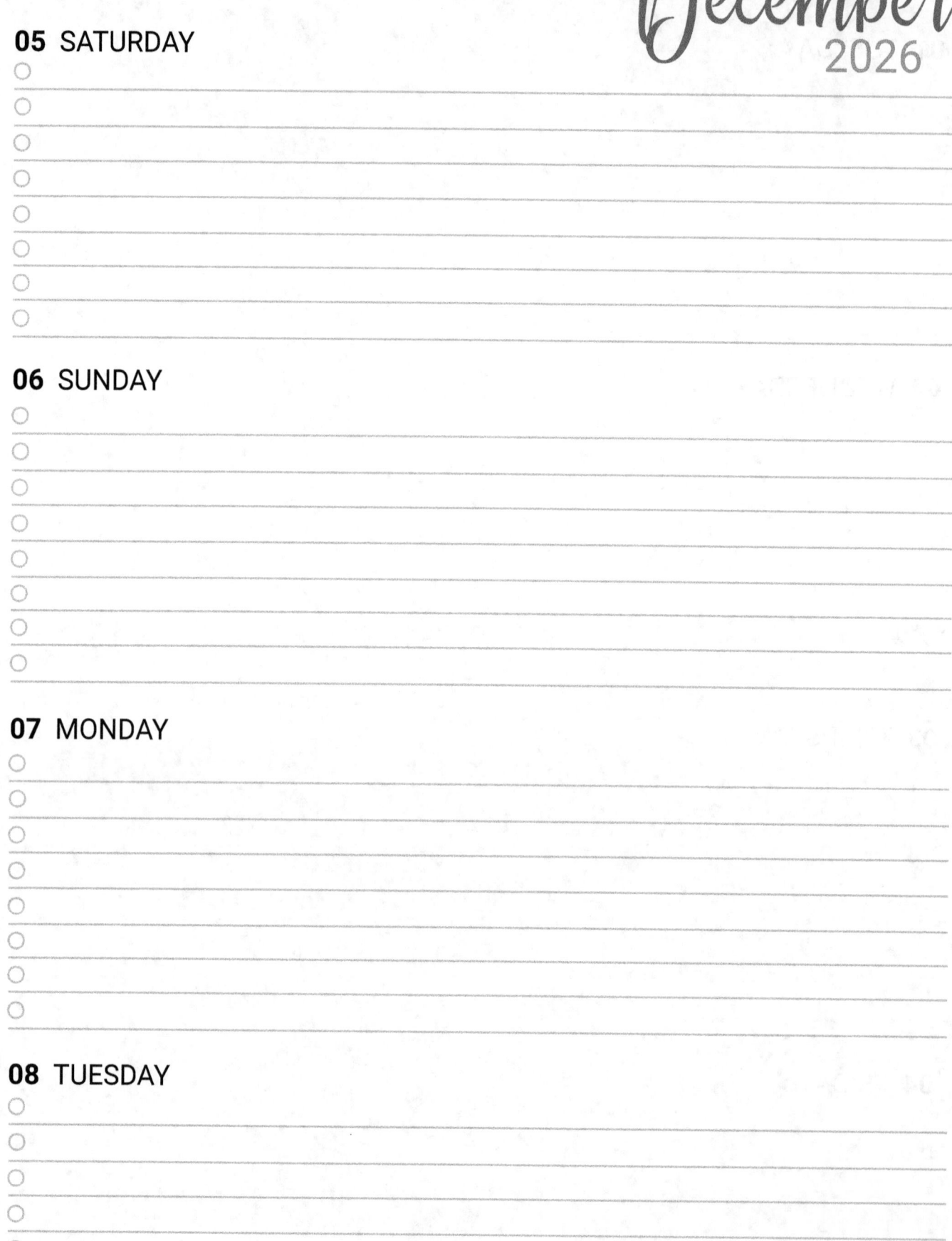

December
2026

05 SATURDAY
○
○
○
○
○
○
○

06 SUNDAY
○
○
○
○
○
○
○
○

07 MONDAY
○
○
○
○
○
○
○
○

08 TUESDAY
○
○
○
○
○

09 WEDNESDAY

10 THURSDAY

11 FRIDAY

12 SATURDAY

13 SUNDAY

14 MONDAY

15 TUESDAY

16 WEDNESDAY

December
2026

17 THURSDAY

18 FRIDAY

19 SATURDAY

20 SUNDAY

21 MONDAY

22 TUESDAY

23 WEDNESDAY

24 THURSDAY

25 FRIDAY

26 SATURDAY

27 SUNDAY

28 MONDAY

29 TUESDAY

30 WEDNESDAY

31 THURSDAY

NOTES

www.ingramcontent.com/pod-product-compliance
Lightning Source LLC
Chambersburg PA
CBHW081332120626
46546CB00011B/3319